The Art of
Muscle
Control

AN INTRODUCTION TO A SPECIALITY
METHOD OF MUSCLE DEVELOPMENT, AND A
MEANS OF ACHIEVING SUPREME
PHYSICAL FITNESS, WITHOUT THE USE OF ANY
APPARATUS WHATSOEVER

By TOM WOODWARD

Edited with additional notes by
Ken Woodward

Illustrated by TONY HOLLAND
Television's "Musical Muscle Man"
Photography by George Greenwood

DISCLAIMER

The exercises and advice contained within this book is for educational and entertainment purposes only. The exercises described may be too strenuous or dangerous for some people, and the reader should consult with a physician before engaging in any of them.

The author and publisher of this book are not responsible in any manner whatsoever for any injury, which may occur through the use or misuse of the information presented here.

The Art of Muscle Control originally published in 1967

PART 1: THE AUTO-RESISTA METHOD

Here is a welcome to you in your aim to achieve and maintain a good physique, and at the same time, to acquire that feeling of being in top-class condition. But before you settle down to training of any kind, do please try to adopt a feeling of happiness and optimism – it means so much towards your success – and I can assure you that almost immediately you will feel that you can become very adept in this fascinating art of muscle control. In fact, your interest will be stimulated right from the first movements.

Do not conjure up any ideas that within a few months you will possess a body like Tony Holland. Yet, in a very short time, you can surprise yourself and your friends by being able to do a few simple movements of muscle control.

Consider first what Tony Holland has done for himself and for those seeking something better in their own physical make-up. I would not try to hide the fact that only a few persons are interested in the big `Mr. Universe` type of physique, and unless they are keenly interested in exceptional physical development, they are inclined to regard this type of physique a freak. Yet, in Tony Holland we have a muscle man who has thrilled the millions of television viewers to such an extend that they eagerly awaited his next appearance. When it was considered that in the TV talent show `Opportunity Knocks,` Tony competed against very talented and experienced artistes from the popular entertainment spheres, one can appreciate what he really has achieved. One of my treasured prizes is one that I won in a similar talent competition many years ago.

The success of Tony Holland offers fine encouragement to those who seek a well-developed body. I like very much his arm pose in Photo 1., because its size looks out of all proportion to his chest and shoulders. Yet, when we look at Photo 2. we get proof that the arms blend in unison with the rest of the body. This is also apparent in

Photos 3, 4 and 5, although the poses are so different. There is something of a clear-defined appearance about Tony's muscular development and, to be quite candid, it could also have an adverse effect on readers because many do not realize what training on progressive lines can do.

Muscle control showmanship is not something new. It was done many years ago by the great Eugen Sandow, and there have been many expert components of the art since then, prominent amongst these being the famous Maxick (who was considered to be probably the first person to make a speciality of this type of routine in his stage act) and the American expert Matysek. I also did muscle control in my own posing act over fifty years ago, and because of my long interest in this particular act, I was delighted to make the acquaintance of Tony Holland, and to congratulate him upon his achievement in introducing the general public once again to the fascination of muscle control.

During Tony's 1965 season at Blackpool, he trained regularly at our health studio, and this gave us several opportunities for discussions on training. Like most of the star athletes, Tony is always willing to give advice to the beginner interested in muscle control and, if you have the opportunity to meet him personally, you will find him to be a charming level-headed person who will be glad to help.

In Photo 2, you can start at the feet and look upwards. You will note that, without being in full contraction, the Lattisimus Dorsi muscles stand out clearly to define a slender waistline. Although Tony has been in training for quite a long while to achieve his physique, he did really start at the bottom of the ladder, and training with weights was an important part of his early training. But, as he desired something more than just big muscles, he found that muscle control was really necessary.

If you have been training on other methods, you will certainly find that a change in routine can work wonders, because from the very first exercise you will feel convinced that you will be able to go through the routine right up to the stage which occupies the mind of expert poseur. Still a better reason for changing to this system is because, after a lengthy training on any particular system of muscle development, the muscles become somewhat bored with the same repetitive movements. If you have been doing heavy weight-training your muscles will naturally be getting tired, so by this control system they are refreshed and stimulated into further action, which usually results in increased muscular development.

Like good feeding, a change is definitely beneficial. In fact it is a necessity. The same thing applies to the mind. Whilst learning the art of muscular contraction and control, you are opening a new field of thought. So therefore that very old saying that a change is as good as a rest is certainly and conclusively proved. I am naturally convinced that those who are new to any kind of physical training will be quite fascinated and eager to go from the contraction and control of one group of muscles to another group with the resulting feeling that their condition of fitness is almost of secondary importance to the thrill of performing these exercises.

You are strongly advised to check up on the notes of breathing. This inhalation and exhalation is a **must** for every exercise, but it is only necessary to expand the chest to its fullest when advised in the instructions.

If you are a beginner in physical training, do not go beyond the instructions. If you have had a fair amount of training on other methods, and you feel sure that your muscles could stand a little extra, you could increase the repetitions and sets, but still do not attempt too many exercises or controls at any time. It is much quicker to master three contractions and controls in one month, than to attempt too many movements without achieving control of any group of muscles to your satisfaction.

This is a six-months Course of Training, but I can assure you that it might well take three years to be in the advanced class similar to

Tony Holland. Even then it is still possible to learn a little more, or to increase the size of the muscles still further.

Both Tony Holland and myself agree that before any progress can be made in the control of the various muscle groups, the muscles must be `felt` when in action. So probably this is just the moment when this should be more fully explained to you . . . and so will you now just give a try-out to the movements commenced on the following page . . .

I wish you every success with your training.

LEARNING MUSCLE CONTROL

It is usual to start with the control of the arm muscles, firstly because these are the quickest to respond to treatment, and also because it is easy to see the effect on these muscles. You may be surprised at the simplicity of these movements, yet they are very important because the same movements that are involved in the very early stages of muscle-control are also the movements which bring about the muscular development and increase in size.

These exercises and movements are so arranged that they must take the beginner by easy stages right up to the standard of the expert performer and, at the same time, provide much information for those who are already familiar with Muscle Control.

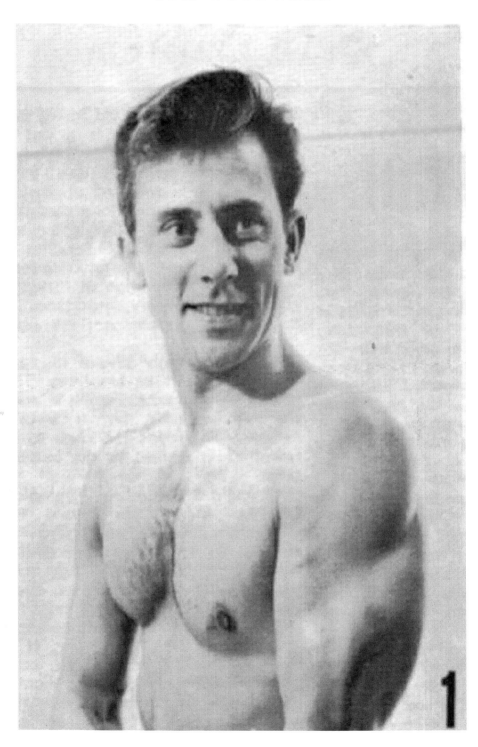

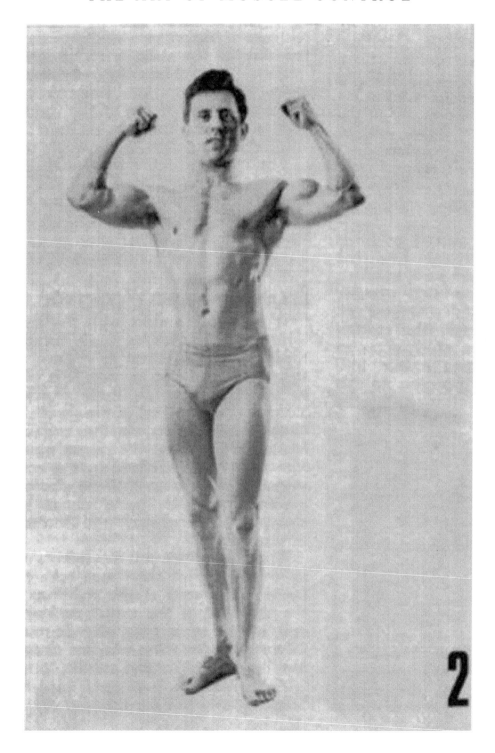

2

TOM WOODWARD

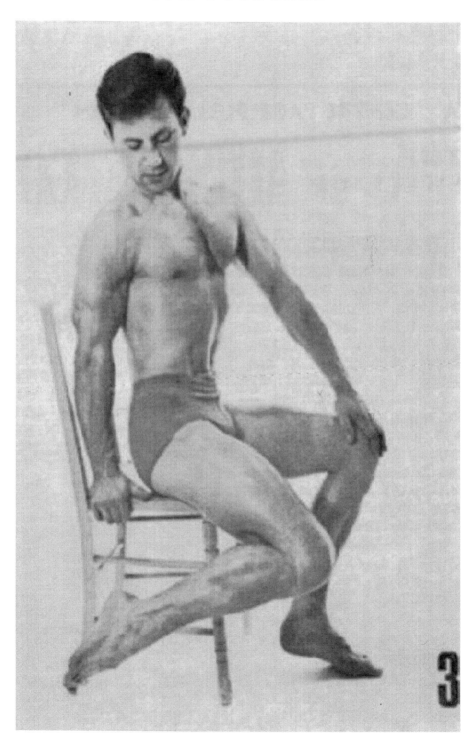

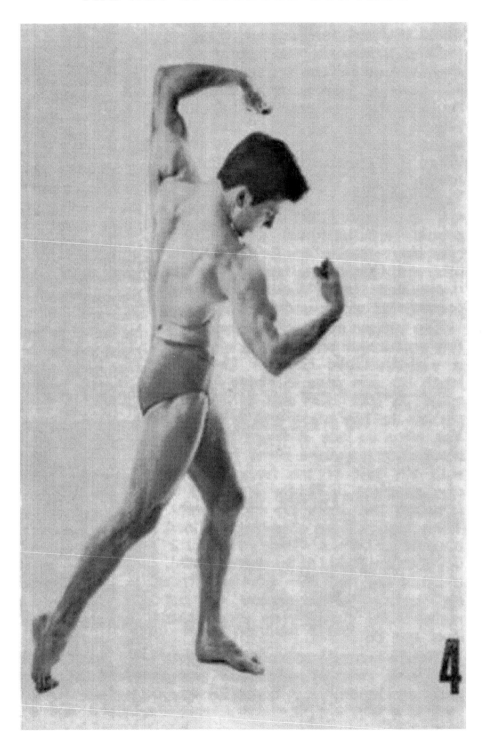

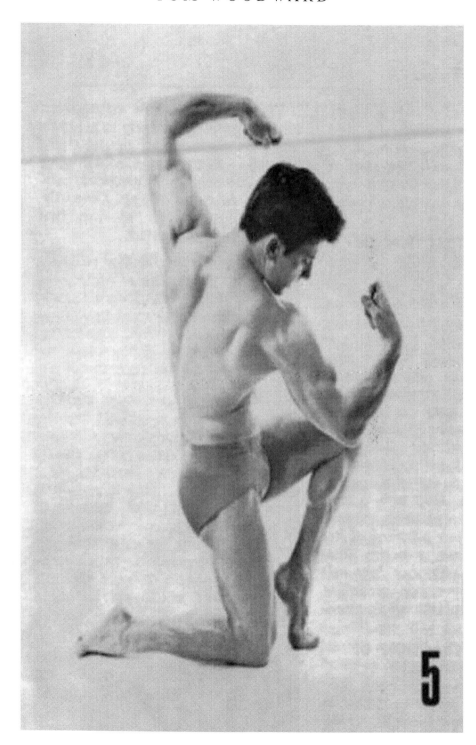

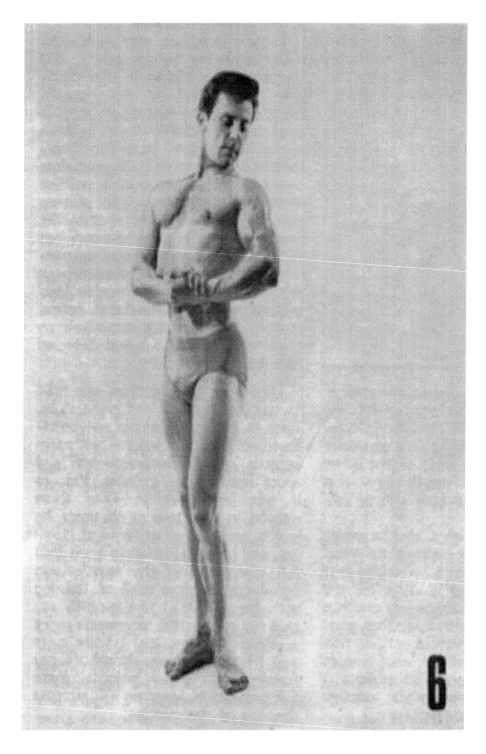

TOM WOODWARD

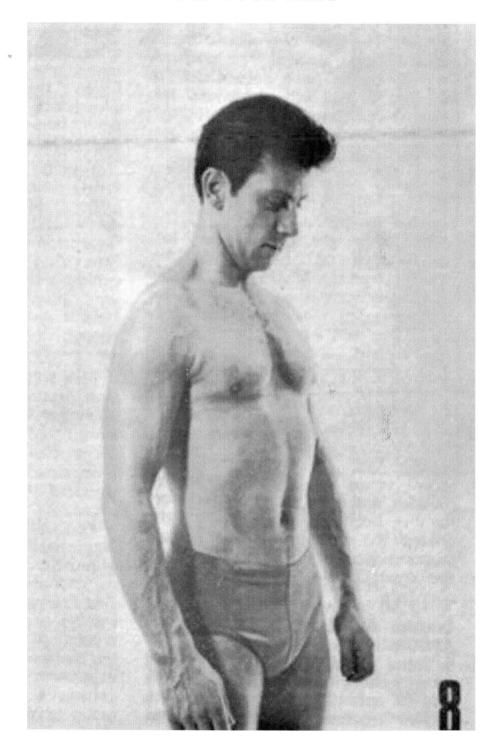

Exercise 1 – CONTRACTION OF THE ARM MUSCLES

Hold your arms down at your sides, slightly bent and away from your body. Close the fists loosely. Inhale and expand your chest to its fullest. Exhale. Then grip the fists again – just a little tighter, count 1 – 2 – 3, and relax. Inhale, exhale, and grip tightly again, even a little tighter than the previous time. Count 1 – 2 – 3, and relax completely.

This is not an exercise for the chest, so do fix your mind on making those forearm and upper arm muscles as hard and as tight as possible. You will also feel a tightening of those muscles on front of the chest (pectorals), but do concentrate on your own arms.

You should now be able to feel and experience the real meaning of muscle contraction. This simple contraction, yet it should be sufficient to convince you that with daily practice you can develop your muscles without expensive equipment. Note carefully that you are advised to inhale and exhale before each contraction movement of this exercise. This is definitely essential, and you will understand why when you come to the full contraction movements.

Exercise 2 – CHEST

Let us now take a look at the chest. If you are conscientiously performing the inhaling and exhaling movements, you are doing much good towards developing the chest in general. The first aim should be to make the chest expand. This produces what is known as a deep chest as in Photo 6. you will understand this better if you compare this photograph with No. 3 which shows the pectoral muscles. These muscles would certainly look out of place if they were over-developed on a flat chest.

Exercise 3 – SHOULDERS

Stand upright, with one foot slightly advanced. Arms at your sides, palms forward. Inhale – exhale. Then raise your arms in an outward and backward movement until they are in line with your shoulders. Pause here. Inhale – exhale – and then raise your arms to full stretch up-wards. Pause – inhale – exhale, and try to reach a little higher. Count 1 – 2 – 3. Relax completely.

If you have done this in the correct manner, you would naturally feel some strain on your abdominal muscles, and as it is usually necessary for the beginner to reduce a little around the waistline, you will begin to experience benefits here right from the start. The next movement will also help . . .

Exercise 4 – WAIST AND ABDOMINALS

Stand upright, feet slightly apart, arms held with the hands at the side of your thighs. (Photo 8). With a slow movement, raise your arms until they are at full stretch upwards. Hold your palms inwards for this movement. Now, with a swing, bend your body forward with the idea of taking your arms between your legs. Return to the arms stretch overhead. Relax completely.

Exercise 5 – CONTRACTOPN OF THE LEG MUSCLES

Stand upright, with your feet slightly apart, and without shoes on your feet – unless the soles of the shoes are very pliable. (I have been amazed when watching persons performing leg exercises whilst, wearing shoes with an almost rigid sole. These hard soles do not give the lower leg muscles free movement in exercising). Stand completely relaxed, then make an effort to grip the floor with your feet. A few attempts will give you the idea of doing this. Grip with a slow deliberate movement which should immediately give you a feeling of leg contraction. Continue with this gripping movement until your legs tell you that they have had sufficient work. Relax. Repeat the whole exercise once only.

Exercise 6 – CONTRACTION OF THE FOREARM MUSCLES

Because you have just given your legs a workout, it would be advisable to perform this next exercise whilst seated. This will give your legs a rest with the chance to recuperate from their efforts. Hold your arms away from your body, fists closed loosely. Bend your arms to bring your forearms almost to right angles with the upper arms, with the palms upwards. Clench the fists tightly and bend your hands inward towards your forearms. Grip tighter. Count 1 – 2 – 3, and relax. Open your hands.

Your gripping movement will commence here. Bend the fingers slowly, gripping all the time, with the fingers apart and with the intention of `squeezing a lemon`. You should now have the feeling of the forearms aching a little. Continue the squeeze until your fists are tightly closed. Hold it until your forearms have had enough, then relax completely.

This will bring you to the end of your first week's training, and I feel sure that you will be already convinced that you can become an expert at muscle control and, at the same time, develop your muscles to such a standard that your body will be admired.

You will note that each exercise is arranged to cover a separate group of muscles, and this is by far the best method of training to adopt for the first four weeks, because you are thus getting a good general idea of what is required in the various actions, how the movements feel and, what is more important, each group of muscles is getting a brief rest whilst another group is in action.

You should liken the arrangement of this Course of Training to a tuition course in commerce or similar study. That is – sections devoted to Beginners, Intermediate, Advanced, and Expertly Advanced stages. Obviously, you are now only at the first beginner's stage of study.

Probably you would like to try a muscle-control movement right now. If so, will you close your fists loosely, grip tightly, and immediately relax the grip. Repeat this a few times, trying to make the gripping and relaxing much quicker each time.

This will see you through the first week of your training, and by the time you get through the complete routine in this Course (which should take you about six months), you should be able to show a surprising change in your physical appearance. Do not make the mistake of trying out the schedule for next week, or next month, before you have accustomed your muscles to cope with the extra demand which will be made upon them.

I know that Tony Holland likes a good workout with a set of weights whenever possible, and he has trained on many occasions at our studio in Blackpool, but all the weight-training methods cannot bring that suppleness of muscle which is necessary for the control work.

There is only one way to become a star performer in any sphere, and that is by specializing in that particular sphere and by doing special exercises with the one single purpose in view. If you are ever able to have a chat with Tony, he will tell you that he has spent many hours before a mirror to achieve a clear outline of the muscle groups. It is possible to arrange two mirrors so that the muscles of the back movements can be watched, and this mirror arrangement will add great interest to your practice because, in addition to feeling and seeing the muscles in action, you can spend a little more time on those muscles which need bringing into line with the others.

Like many other artistes who have to tour the theatres and night clubs, Tony found that it was not convenient to travel a set of weights with him because of the inconvenience and space required for training. Yet, as it was imperative to keep those muscles in good trim at all times, he had to resort to other forms of training, and I was delighted to know that full contraction of the muscles was his choice. After a spell of training with the weights. I can honestly say that full contraction movements make a relaxing change, and I know quite well that even if you do not do any training with heavy weights, these full contraction exercises will increase the size of the muscles.

PART 2: MORE EXERCISES FOR
THE SECOND WEEK OF YOUR TRAINING

We can now commence on the schedule for the second week, and now you will begin to realize what progressive training really means. When you attempt these movements, you should be aware that it is necessary to inhale and exhale at the commencement of each contraction.

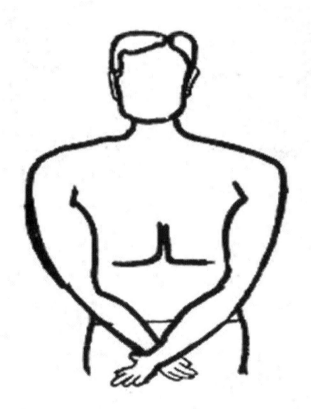

Check up on the inhaling and exhaling advice and do not at any time do any particular movement whilst holding your breath. This will impede progress.

KEY EXERCISE

This exercise could mean so much to your success. In fact, it could be the secret of many advanced controls. We can start with exercise 1, making first a full contraction of the legs (as advised in Ex. 5). Inhale, exhale, and then repeat Exercise 1, doing a full contraction of the arms. Inhale, exhale, then inhale again, and expand your chest to its fullest by raising it and pushing it forward. Keep the legs contracted whilst contracting the arm muscles, and then keep the leg and arm muscles contracted whilst expanding the chest.

Exercise 7 – BICEPS

Stand as in Exercise 1, grip the fists tightly and slowly bend your arms until your hands touch the shoulders. Count 1 – 2 – 3. Lower your arms and repeat. Three repetitions in all. This now brings us back to the next movement . . . which is for the back muscles.

Exercise 8 – SHOULDERS AND BACK

Stand upright, feet slightly apart. Hands in front of your thighs, with the right hand grasping the thumb of the left hand. This will bring the fingers of the left hand on the outside of the right hand. Grip the hands tightly and slowly raise the arms forward until they are at full stretch upwards. (See photo 7). Move the arms slowly, and pull hard on the hands. Inhale. Exhale . Try to reach a little higher. Count 1 – 2 – 3. Keep pulling hard and, still pulling, bend the arms to bring the hands behind the head. Straighten the arms upwards again, then lower them to the starting position, still pulling hard all the time. Relax.

Exercise 9 – CHEST (Pectorals)

Stand as illustrated in Photo 8, chest raised. Bring the hands slowly inwards, at the same time pressing your upper arms under those muscles in front of your chest. Continue the movement of the arms until you can cross your wrists together in front of your body. (See illustration). Keep the arms straight and try to make those chest muscles feel like little hard lumps. You might get a better feeling if you turned your palms inwards. When the wrists are crossed, straighten your arms downwards and raise your chest a little more. Count 1 – 2 – 3. Relax and repeat. Three repetitions in all.

To continue our routine for this week, and to give the upper body a slight rest, we will proceed with a leg exercise.

Exercise 10 – LEG MUSCLES

Place one hand upon an object, to act as a support for maintaining your balance. Raise one foot forward, as in Photo 9. Point the toes forward, then inward, trying to make all the leg muscles feel tight and hard. Count 1 – 2 – 3. With the toes still pointing forward, move the leg slowly to bring it to the position shown in Photo 10. Repeat the moving of the foot to bring the toes inwards again, trying to make all the leg muscles feel hard. Repeat.

Exercise 11 – ABDOMINALS

Now is the time to pay some attention once again to the abdominal region, and for this exercise you will lie face upwards on the floor. Much will depend upon the condition of your waistline when doing these movement. They seem very simple, but a little too much enthusiasm can bring about a very painful feeling for a few days afterwards, so do go easy with this movement just now.

The idea of this exercise is to pull your stomach muscles (abdominals) inwards as much as possible. Relax, then repeat. This is sufficient unless your abdominal muscles are in good condition.

Exercise 12 – NECK

Whilst on the floor from the previous exercise, you can try a neck exercise. Interlace your fingers, and place your hands underneath the back of your head. Raise the head to bring your chin in towards your chest. Relax. Lower head and repeat.

This will now complete your second week of training, and I feel sure that you will not be getting an eager feeling to travel much faster with your training, but it is still very necessary to curb over enthusiasm. During the third week, we shall step up the training a little more.

THIRD AND FOURTH WEEKS
Exercise 13 – BICEPS

You will commence this exercise with your arms held out sideways in line with your shoulders. Clench your fists tightly, and slowly bend your arms to bring them to the position shown in Photo 2. Pause. Inhale, then exhale, still keeping your biceps muscles hard. Grip your fists tighter still to make your biceps muscles swell just a little more. Count 1 – 2 – 3, then relax. Straighten your arms and repeat.

Now you can try an actual muscle control movement here. Go to the position shown in Photo 2. Keep the muscle quite hard and turn the palms forwards as in Photo 11. Turn them inwards again. Do this movement alternately for a few times and notice how your muscles move about. This movement is to produce that suppleness which is necessary for the advanced controls.

Exercise 14 – BACK

For the back muscles again, you will repeat Exercise 8, already described. When the hands are lowered to the position behind the head, you will pull hard and make a circular movement with your shoulders, bringing them close to your ears and then taking them backwards, at the same time keeping the elbows well outward to make a large full circle. Do this for a couple of times, and then reverse the direction. You should now feel that you have more muscles in your back than you realized. Straighten your arms upward, whilst pulling hard. Relax now, ready for–

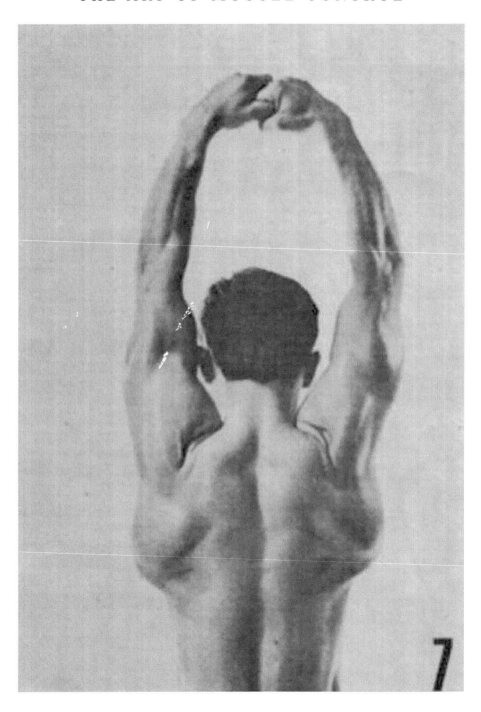

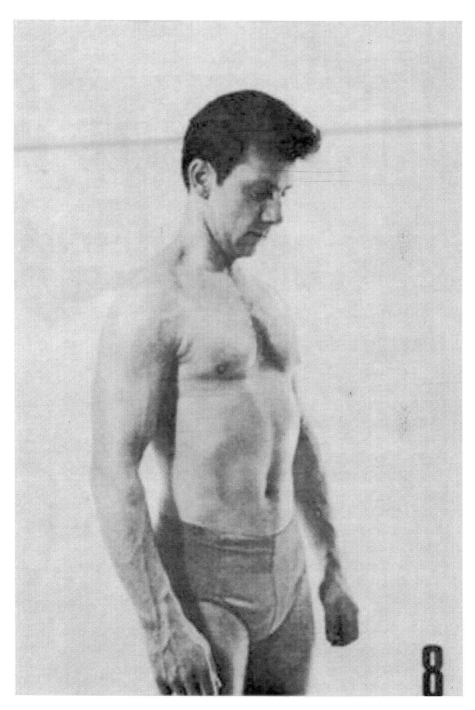

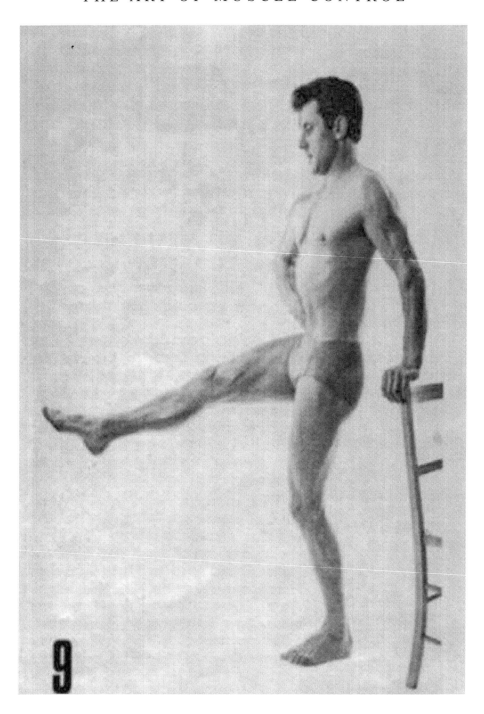

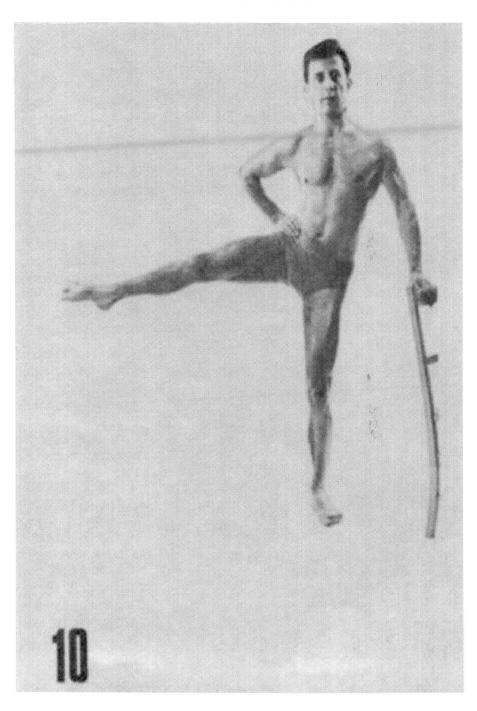

10

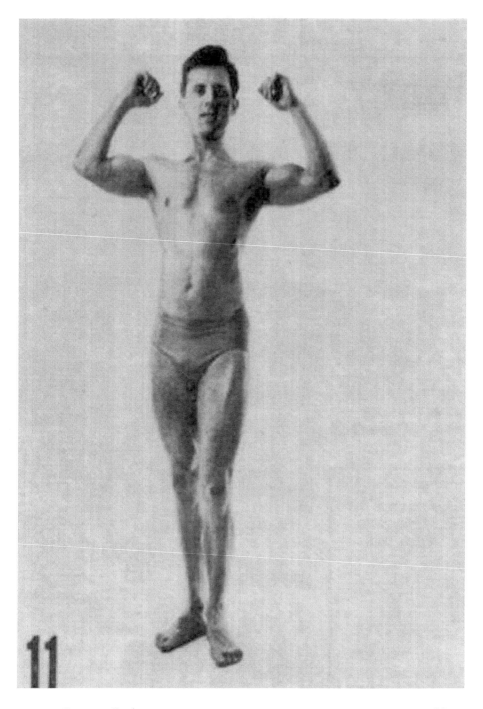

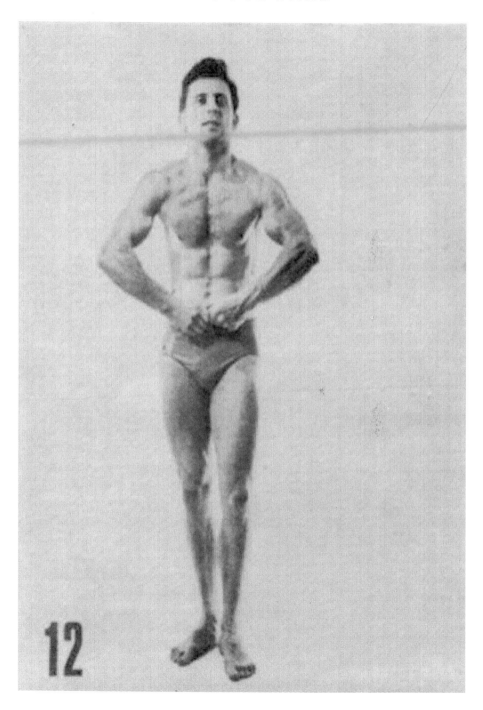

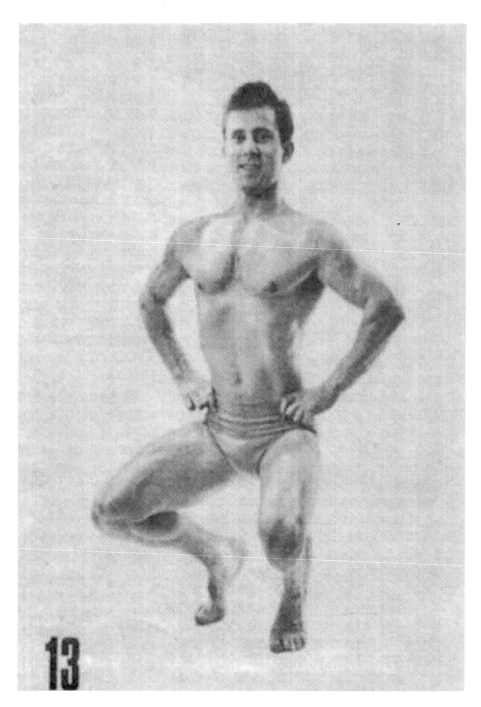

Exercise 15 – CONTROL OF THE PECTORAL MUSCLE

After repeating Exercise 9 a few times as already described, you can grasp your hands together (grip as for Ex. 9) with the hands held away from the body and in front of the waist. Bend forward slightly, as shown in Photo 12. Now, by pulling and relaxing the thumbs, you can make the pectoral muscles jump about. It is now up to you to perfect the correct position by performing this movement in front of a mirror. If your hands are a little too high, they will hide the chest muscles. If they are a little too low, you will not get a good effect of the control. This also applies to the forward leaning – you must bend at just the right angle to get the near perfect effect.

When you are satisfied that you have the right position, you should increase the power and speed of the jerks on your thumb. I feel sure that this will convince you that simple movements can bring effective results. It takes a good performer to hold his body as Tony Holland does in Photo 12, and to perform these controls. You will find it much easier by leaning forward a little more at first.

Exercise 16 – LEGS

This exercise will now bring the legs into action. Stand upright, with your feet about twelve inches apart. Raise your heels off the floor as high as possible. Lower your heels to the floor, and repeat. When you can control your balance whilst standing on your toes, you will bend your legs to the squat position as shown in Photo 13. Straighten your legs upwards and repeat. Each day you should try to go a little lower until you are eventually sitting on your heels. This is known as the 'deep squat'. These squatting movements should be done with speed, unless you desire to increase the size of this area. When the deep squat is done slowly it has a tendency to increase the size of the hips and buttocks, which is not often required. When done with speed you can usually reduce any surplus weight in this region.

You can now finish this session by sitting on the chair in the position shown in Photo 3. Place the legs in a similar position, with the toes of one foot resting on the floor. The idea now is to raise your heel and bring your calf muscle into tight contraction. Lower the knee and repeat a few times.

Going back to the closing paragraphs of the introductory chapter, you will recall that I stated that the muscles must be 'felt' when in action. This really means that you must be able to contract any group of muscles in action. You must be able to do so by will-power alone. This is definitely a case of the mind controlling the muscles. In many cases control of the muscles really means alternately contracting and relaxing the group in action. It is necessary to move the limbs when doing some controls, others should be done without any limb movement. So do make sure that you are able to fully contract any group of muscles before you attempt the control movements. This is the way to success in muscle control.

There are only two real secrets of success in this fascinating branch of physical training. One is conscientiousness in practice, following instructions, and curbing of your enthusiasm to travel too quickly. The second essential is that when doing the contraction movements, the muscles must be forced to their limits. This advice will be repeated often.

If, in addition to muscle control, muscle development is also needed, commence again at Exercise 1, and repeat each exercise. This will make two 'sets'

PART 3: THE SECRET OF SUCCESS

We now come to the most vital part of the training for muscle control. There is only one way by which the controls can be mastered, and that is by concentration. You have so far been shown a few movements which lay the foundations for the advanced controls, and it is now really a case of mind over matter – for you have to learn to move any group of muscles about at your command.

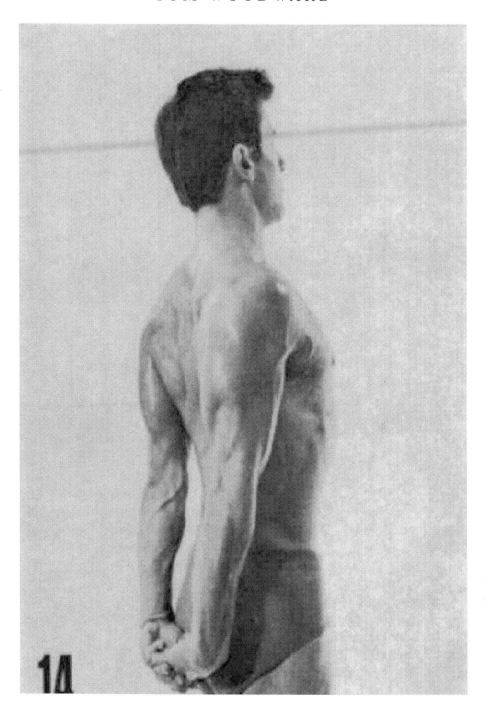

14

THE ART OF MUSCLE CONTROL

If Tony Holland is appearing on television, or in a show n your neighbourhood, I strongly advise you to watch his performance as often as you can. If it is possible for you to meet hm, I am sure that you will learn a great deal, for Tony is always willing t o assist anyone who is keenly interested in mastering this delicate form of physical training. When I was learning muscle posing, I would make a habit of watching all others, and try to memorize a little on each occasion.

You will only accomplish this perfection of mind over matter by concentrating your mind on the group of muscles in action when performing any of the contraction movements already described. You already have a fair idea of what is required in these movements, and when you come to the full contraction movements you will need to concentrate more than ever on what you are doing.

At this stage of your training, you will still have some control movements which depend upon the movement of the limbs and joints, but when watching Tony Holland in performance, you should take particular notice that there is no movement of anything but the specific group of muscles. These are the advanced controls of the experts.

Going back to my own early days, I recall the great Eugen Sandow, whose name was a household word, and who was the idol of all interested in physical culture. Sandow's mastery over muscle control enabled him to work different groups of muscles simultaneously, and after a long period of practice, I mastered this technique. I could control and manipulate the biceps of one arm, the triceps of the other arm, the calf of one leg, and the thigh of the other leg – all at same time – with all these muscle groups dancing in time to the music played for my act. This will emphasize to you why I am particularly keen to stress that mind-over matter is a most important part of physical training.

In this course, I will bring you to this stage of muscle-control perfection if you will keep to the training, but I can assure you that you must be able to understand the meaning of full contraction and have your muscles sufficiently well developed. When doing the arm contraction of Exercise 1 and the bicep contraction of Exercise 13, you must take those muscles as hard and as large as possible by gripping and relaxing the fists in jerky movements. The same thing applies to all other muscle groups also. There is no magic way – only hard practice.

When performing a movement for the second time, it is termed a repetition movement. When this repetition has been twice or more times, it comprises a "set". The terms "repetitions" and "sets" will be brought into future routines. Each training spell you do is referred to as a "session".

To finish off your training for the first month, you could add one or more repetitions to each set of repetitions already advised for the exercises. At present do not perform too many repetitions – just sufficient to make you feel that you have had a good workout on each set. In the schedule for your second month, you will be given more strenuous movements and also a combination of two or more movements. The fact that you have to study the instructions for each movement takes time, but when you know the movements quite well, you will be amazed at how little time it takes to reach the stage of advanced controls. If your time is limited, you should concentrate on any group of muscles which you feel needs improvement.

GENERAL HINTS

I am somewhat amused when I read a certain number of repetitions being advised for each exercise. I know quite well that each individual needs a slightly different routine as regards repetition work. I like to leave it to each pupil to do what is considered by himself to be the most suitable. I offer guidance about not overdoing any exercise until the muscles have been trained to cope with the extra efforts they may be asked to take, but I do strongly advise each pupil to make sure that there is an improvement each day in some respect, no matter how little it may seem to be. Make a habit of trying to get an all-round increase in your measurements but, and this is a strong "but", do not try too many exercises at one session. Make a practice of giving three groups of muscles a real thorough workout for a month, then, if you have time, you could do a little for the other groups. Trying to get an all-around increase at the same time is like trying to be a champion athlete in a number of events. By doing this you will become fair at them all, but not very good at any one.

Make your arms, chest, and abdominals, or any other three groups, the main training for a month or so, then it will only take a few contractions to keep them in trim whilst you concentrate on three different groups for the next month. This way will be far the quickest.

The reason why the number of repetitions cannot be fixed the same for all is because some persons can take much more exercise before getting tired and also possess the power to recuperate quickly. Again some days it is possible to do a little extra, whilst on other occasions the muscles will only take less repetitions.

If you wish to rapidly increase the size of your muscles, you should give them a good workout. Do a few movements on other groups of muscles. This will give the first group a rest. Commence again with the first group and give them another workout, this will make another set. I can honestly promise you that if your biceps are measured before and after two sets, you will find an increase. This has been proved by many who have had the idea that they had reached their limit after a course of weight training. Do the 1, 2 and 3 sets routine for a month, then give them a rest except for bringing them into action in your posing routine. Keep your training going by using the same method on some other groups.

This piece of advice may surprise you. You will notice that some movements can be done whilst seated, such as the arms, shoulders and neck. This will be all to your benefit because it will conserve energy, more so after a workout on the legs. I learned the value of this in my early days of training, whilst being tired after being on my feet all day at work.

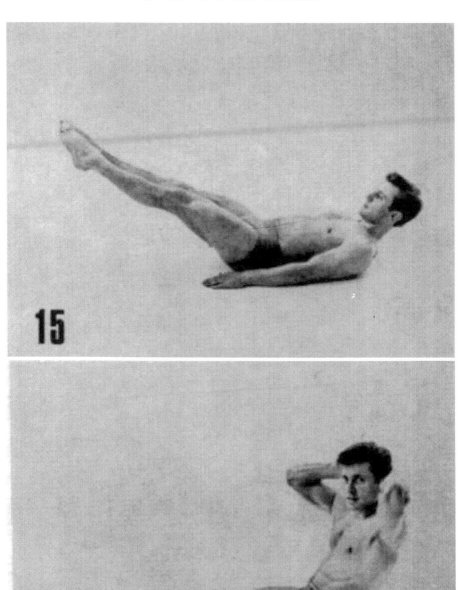

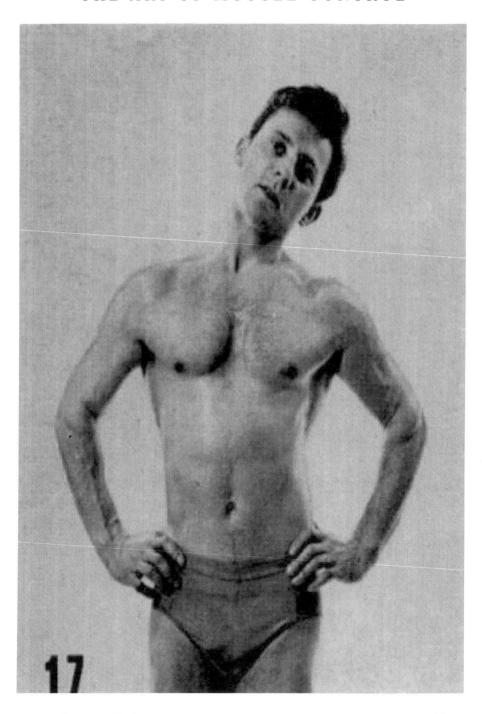

17

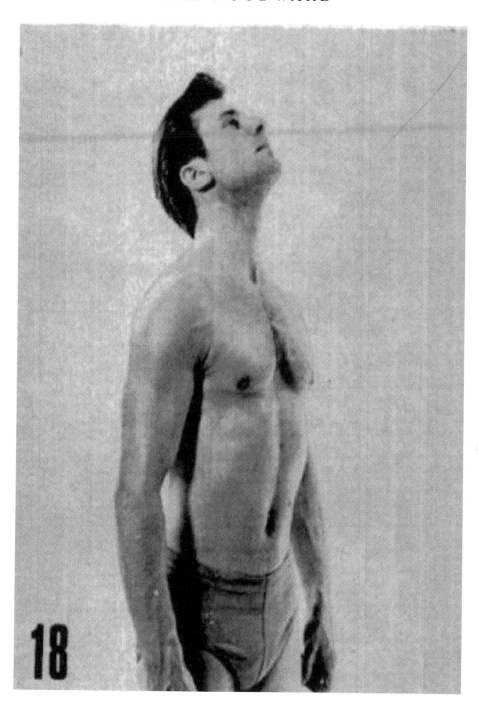

18

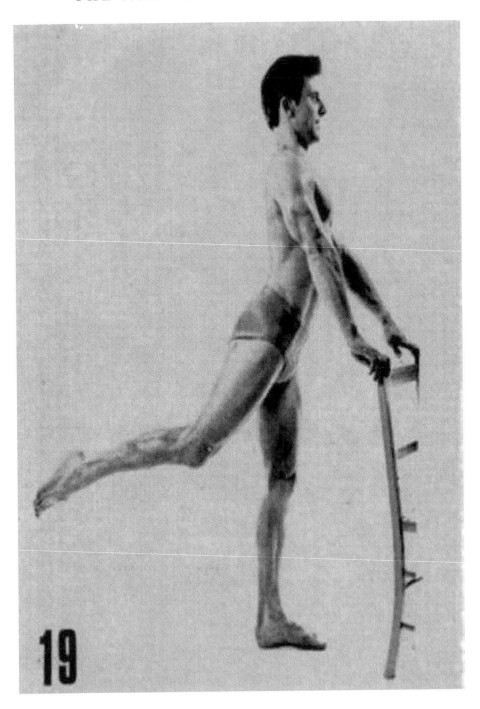

19

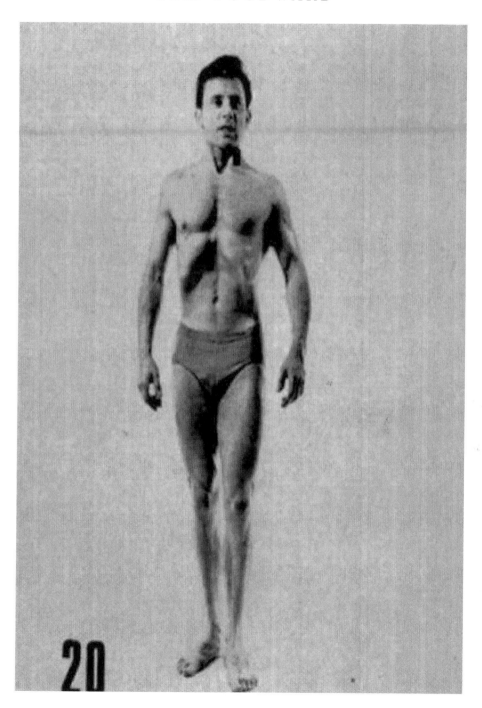

THE ART OF MUSCLE CONTROL

Do not have any doubts about losing size of your muscles whilst resting. It is recognized by many athletic coaches that when muscles are developed they will keep their tone and size for a fair length of time.

If you do not wish for exceptional muscular development, you could spread your training over more groups. After a good workout for a week or so, take a rest for a day to give your muscles a chance to recuperate from the exertions placed upon them. When you read again through the instructions for the various exercises and controls, you will find many items of advice, some of which are repeated to assist in making quick progress.

I can honestly assure you that if you practice with the idea of making progress, it is impossible not to do so. So do be fair to yourself and practice conscientiously. Do not try to learn all the exercises for development and control within a few weeks. This is arranged as a six month course, but you will find sufficient variations to last you for three years, and then probably you will still not be as good as you would like to be.

When doing the suggested "count", you could do so under your breath. There is no need to do it audibly. Increase the count from three upwards to fit in with your progress.

SECOND MONTH
INTERMEDIATE CLASS

We will commence the schedule for the second month with another arm-development movement, but this time it is for the muscles at the back of the upper arm, the triceps muscles. The reason why Tony's upper arm is so pronounced in Photo 1 is because the triceps muscle has been developed up to the same standard as the biceps muscle. This is one of the secrets of developing large upper-arms.

Exercise 17 – TRICEPS

Stand as in Photo 14, with the fingers interlaced tightly. Straighten your arms, and pull hard with your hands. At the same time, move them slightly away from the body. Relax the fingers, then repeat. After the first week, you can grip tightly, then bend your arms slightly. Pull hard and straighten the arms. Repeat. You should now feel the triceps muscles getting very hard indeed.

Exercise 18 – ABDOMINALS
LEG RAISING

You will lie on the floor, face upwards, with your hands at your sides, as in Photo 15. Raise your feet off the floor, keeping your toes pointed forward and your legs straight. Raise them, if possible to the height shown in Photo 15. Replace feet on the floor and repeat. When you are able to do this fairly easily, you will raise your feet a little higher, until they are at right angles with your upper body. It might take you a few weeks before you can accomplish this.

Exercise 19 – ABDOMINALS
BODY RAISING

For this next movement, it is usual to place the feet under some heavy article, but I can allow a little cheating for your first attempts at this. Lie flat on the floor with your head resting in your hands, and now raise the upper body off the floor as in Photo 16. If you have difficulty in doing this, you could raise your buttocks off the floor, then return them to the floor, and at the same time, sit up. It will be a big help if you can do the dropping of the buttocks and raising of the body in one movement. Go very steady at first with these leg and body- raising movements, but when your muscles will stand it, increase by one repetition in each day until you can do each one six times. The movement should really be performed slowly, but you may do them with speed just now, then gradually work towards the slower movement, which calls for more contraction effort.

It would be foolish to develop a good upper body without developing the neck to the same standard so now onto. . .

Exercise 20 – NECK STRETCHING

Stand upright, in an easy manner. Bend the head sideways, as in Photo 17. Move the head to the right and left alternately. As you stretch one side of the neck, you will be contracting the muscles on the opposite side. The more effort put into the stretch will mean more contraction. Two repetitions will suffice at first. This could be followed with a forward bend, as in Photo 8. Bring the chin as near to the chest as possible, then take the head backwards as far as possible, as in Photo 18.

Before going to the more advanced work, you can now devote some time to testing yourself. Start with Exercise 1, and add one or more repetitions to each movement, doing them so that you must force the muscles to perform the last repetition each time. If you work up to four repetitions and feel like adding another one, then your concentration has not been sufficient. At the end of the third repetition, you should feel as though you have had enough. This is the time when the muscles must be forced to do another repetition. When a muscle aches in this manner, it is growing, and just a little more expansion at this time will increase its size.

After giving one set of muscles a thorough work-out, it is advisable to change to another set which will enable the first muscle group to recuperate. Repeat this process with all the exercises you have mastered.

To explain what is meant by forcing those muscles, let me refer to the training of runners, if they did not force themselves to run faster during their training, they would never reach the record-breaking stage. Again, if weightlifters did not force themselves to lift a pound or two extra, they would never break records. In many instances it is necessary to coax the muscles for a supreme effort, but if they have not been trained to do that little bit extra, they cannot respond when called upon.

Another very special reason for full contraction is because the blood is thus squeezed from the muscles, and on relaxation a supply of new blood is attracted, and naturally the circulation is benefited in this manner.

Not to get back to the remainder of the schedule.

After a few repetitions of exercise 10, the leg can be raised backwards as in Photo 19. Lower to the floor and repeat.

You will need a little suppleness in the leg muscles, so stand upright with one leg bent backwards, and with the heel almost touching the buttocks. Do a few sharp, jerky kicks until you can feel the muscles at the back of the thigh (the hamstring group – biceps femoris, etc.) aching a little.

Now sit down and raise one foot off the floor and work the foot in a circular movement. You can now feel the calf muscles in action.

This brings us to the waist region once more, and if you have got your waist into a reasonable shape, you can consider this abdominal control movement.

Exercise 21

Stand upright, as in Photo 20. Draw your Abdomen inwards as far as possible. The movement on the floor, in Exercise 11, should have prepared you for this. When the abdomen is well in, inhale, exhale, and do try to pull it in a little more. You could assist this pull in by a little pressure from your hands. Relax, and let the abdomen fall outwards again. Repeat. This is necessary to prepare your body for the Abdominal Isolation – The Rope – as it is named.

You could get much benefit from this movement if you made a

habit of doing a little massage of the abdomen. A chapter on massage will be included later, but a daily rub, in a circular movement, with your bare hands, could get some of the flesh away and, at the same time, tone up the muscles.

I take it that you now still wish to excel in muscle control, so you can now continue with the schedule for the third month, but I can assure you that these exercises will now test your muscles to the limit and even then you should still try to get a little more out of them. It is not a good literary style to repeat advice like this, but your success really does depend upon doing it just a little better than others can do it.

I shall now deal with the method of achieving the best development of the various muscle groups.

Commence with **Exercise 1.**

Grip the fists tightly. Bend the arms a little. Pause. Inhale, exhale. Grip tighter to increase the contraction. Count 1-2-3. Move the arms a little more towards your shoulders. Pause again, and increase the power of contraction. Count 1-2-3. Move the hands to touch the shoulders. Pause. Grip tightly. Force the biceps to swell a little more. Count 1-2-3. Pause. Inhale, exhale. Contract a little more, again counting 1-2-3. Hold this, then count 1-2-3-4-5-6, increasing the contraction at each count.

Immediately take your arms to the position in Photo 14, which is the triceps contraction exercise, and now give the triceps a thorough test on the 1-2-3-4-5-6 idea described above.

You should now be ready for a good workout on the chest, as in Exercise 9, doing the 1-2-3-4-5-6 contractions. In fact, you should now work on all muscle groups in this style, because this will definitely increase the size of the muscles and, at the same time, bring about a clear muscular definition, which is most important.

TOM WOODWARD

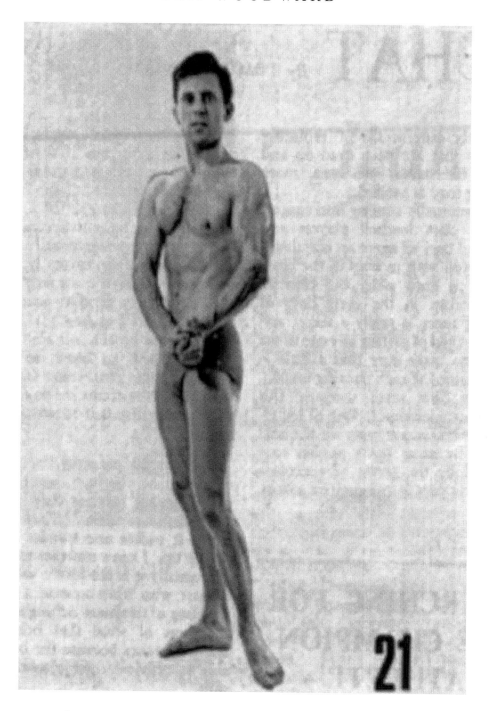

PART 4: THE THIRD MONTH OF YOUR TRAINING

This brings me now to the third month, which is now definitely arranged to give a special touch to your training. It does not mean that you can finish your training at this stage. Tony Holland would soon convince you that it takes more like three years than three months to become an expert at muscle control, but this system of training is arranged on similar lines to our tuition in handbalancing and acrobatics. In this branch of our postal service we have trained pupils who were able to give a very good display (in fact many have won top prizes in variety competitions in the theatres), after only three months of tuition, but they realized that it takes a very long time to master some of the stunts which should enable them to appear at first-class theatres and circuses. Yet the fact remains that once they have appeared in public and received good appreciation for their display, it increases their keenness to get to the top. I feel convinced that the same thing applies to muscle control, but the greatest prize to be won is that feeling of fitness and knowing the secret of how to keep it.

We will start off this month with the Auto-Resista movements. This is a name I give to a system of muscle-building where one group of muscles provides the resistance for building up another group. This is the theme behind all methods of training with appliances. The same principle is applied here as in weight-training, but instead of increasing the poundage of the weights, you provide your own increased resistance. This really means that this system is adaptable for the weakest and also for the strongest person, because weak persons cannot strain themselves and the strongest can regulate the amount of resistance which is needed to extend any group of muscles to its limit.

As at the beginning of the Course, we will commence again with the arm muscles, because the movements here can be explained more fully and made easier to understand.

Exercise 22 – CURL RESISTANCE MOVEMENT

Stand upright, with the left hand in front of the left thigh. Place your right hand on top, with the thumb on the outside of your left thumb. Grip the hands similar to shaking hands, as in Photo 21. You will bring the left hand towards your shoulder, with the arm bent, resisting the rising of the left hand by pressing against it with the right hand (see Photo 6). Use just enough resistance to make your left arm vibrate slightly. When the hands are against the shoulders, make an extra effort and count 1 – 2 – 3. Repeat. Then change the position of the hands.

Exercise 23 – PECTORALS

Grasp hands, hold them in front of your chest, with the arms bent – upper arms at the sides of the chest. You will now grip your hands tightly and try to make the elbows touch – at the same time lowering your hands a little. Keep the chest raised high throughout the whole movement. When the pectorals are fully flexed, do the counting and force them a little more. Relax, then repeat.

Exercise 24

Your next movement is for the shoulders. Stand, with your hands in front of your shoulders, palms upward. Now imagine that you are holding a heavy bar in your hands. Raise your elbows. You will now do the "barbell press", taking your hands slightly outward whilst they are going up. Make this imaginary bar feel as if you have to use all your strength to move it. When the arms are straight up above your body, relax, then repeat.

You will now feel like taking a rest, so onto the floor for. . .

Exercise 25

Lie on the floor, face upwards, with a pillow upon which to rest your head. Place your hands on the floor behind your shoulders, palms downward. Take your weight on your hands and head whilst raising your shoulders off the floor. This is known as the "Wrestler's Bridge" position. It might take you a couple of weeks before you can hold the position as Tony does in Photo 22. Unless you have done this exercise previously, you are strongly advised to do it once only until your neck can bear the weight easily. I consider this exercise to be a re-vitaliser of the nervous system and it is probably one reason why wrestlers can carry on with their contests at an age when most competitive athletes have retired from active sport.

Whilst on the floor, you could now try an advanced and rather strenuous abdominal exercise. . .

Exercise 26

Start as in Exercise 18, but raise the feet only a few inches off the floor. Hold this position and count 1 – 2 – 3. Raise the feet a little higher, count three again, and so on until the legs are upwards and at right angles to the body. Make about six pauses on the way up, and the same number on the way down. The reason for these stops is to make the abdominal muscles do the work of raising the feet and of resisting the downward pull. When you get to the stage when this is somewhat easy, you could try to repeat the movement by taking the feet wide apart whilst raising them and bringing them together at right angles to the body. Split the legs apart again whilst lowering them. This will help you to get that ribbed appearance of the abdomen.

We could now also try a resistance exercise for the legs whilst lying down. . .

Exercise 27

Still lying, raise the feet about twelve inches or so off the floor, the insides of the feet touching each other, but with the knees wide apart and with the legs slightly bent. You will press the feet against each other and, at the same time, place your thoughts on squeezing something almost solid between your legs. Make the resistance just enough to force all your thigh muscles into action. Hold this squeezing movement until your knees are touching each other. Repeat. Then do the same pressing movement with your feet but, this time, bend your legs to bring your heels in towards your buttocks. Straighten the legs out whilst still squeezing. This will give your calf muscles something to do.

PART 5: CONCLUDING THE THIRD MONTH OF TRAINING
Exercise 28

You can now stand up again to finish off with a resistance movement for the triceps muscles. Stand as shown in Photo 14, with the hands changed over into this position, fists closed loosely, palms outward, thumbs and fingers touching. Bend the arms slightly. Imagine that you have a piece of steel in your hands which needs bending. Slowly work the hands around until all the fingers are touching. When the backs of the fingers of each hand are touching, count $1 - 2 - 3$, then give an extra pull by straightening your arms and pushing the fingers together.

Exercise 29 – ABDOMINAL CONTRACTION

You can now try the full contraction of the abdominal muscles. This will definitely prove the value of keeping the waist-line in condition.

Stand upright, with the hands flat and placed on the back of your buttocks. Lean forward just enough to create a droop in your shoulders. You are now ready for the contraction movement.

You may have to do a little thinking for yourself, and yet the instructions are definitely clear. You will now slide your hands slowly downwards, pressing on your buttocks whilst doing so. The idea is to make your body feel a little shorter, but without actually leaning forward. You will certainly get the feeling of your abdominal muscles getting cramped together. When you feel them hardening, hold it whilst

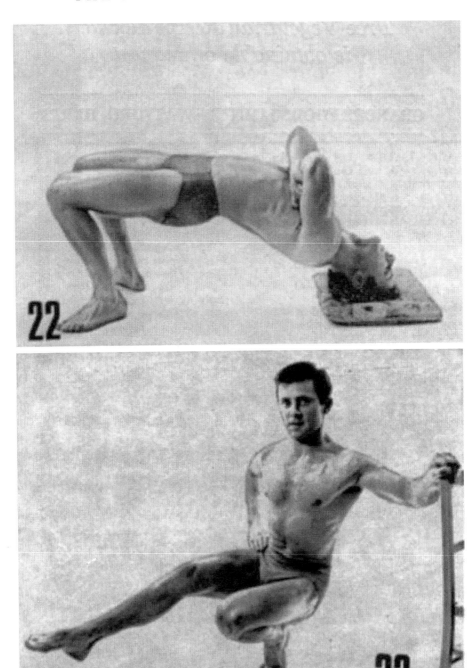

doing the count. Relax completely. Inhale, – exhale. Then pull in your abdominal muscles. Keep the abdomen in this position. Inhale, – exhale, and pull it in just a little more. Hold it again. Inhale, – exhale, and still force it inwards a little more. Then repeat the contraction movements.

This will prepare you for that fascinating abdominal control movement called the "Rope".

But ow, for the time being, take a rest from this exercise by doing a lifting movement known as. . . "Lateral Raise". . .

Exercise 30

Stand easy, with your arms at your sides, palms outwards. Now imagine that you are pulling against a strong spring which is testing you severely. Make the movement slowly until the arms are in line with the shoulders. Take the arms backwards whilst raising them. When in line with your shoulders, turn the palms forward and pull hard until your arms are at full stretch in front of your chest. Whilst doing this pull, you will stretch your arms as much as possible. When the hands are together in front of your chest, inhale – exhale, then take your arms backwards again, pulling hard at the "spring" whilst doing so.

Exercise 31

The legs are now ready for attention, and this will probably be your most difficult exercise. Place your hand on a support, and go down to the deep squat position. Steady yourself, and try to raise one foot off the floor as in Photo 23. Practice this until it feels quite easy to do with either leg. This will certainly give your leg muscles something to do. When you can do this, you will be very eager to stand on one foot and do a deep-knee bend as in the photograph. . . This will now bring us to Muscle Control proper. . . for the following part of the Course.

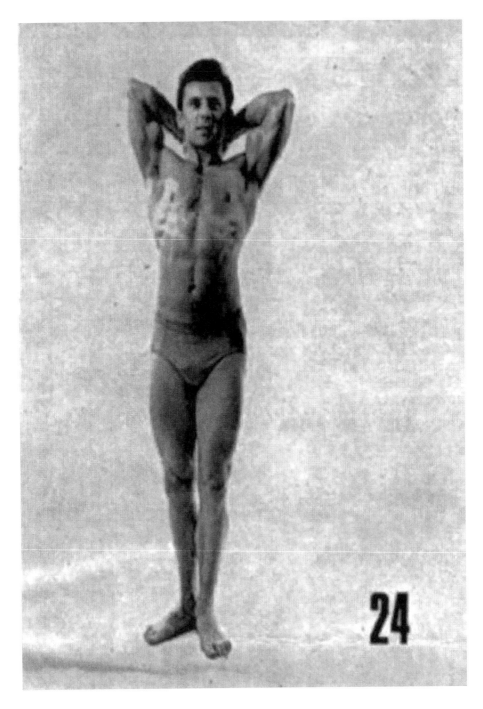

PART 6: MUSCLE CONTROL MOVEMENTS FOR THE FOURTH MONTH
Exercise 32

As usual, we will commence with the upper arms. Hold the arms as in Photo 2 position. Contract and relax the biceps muscles by quick jerks of the hands. Increase the speed of these for a number of times. Then do the same thing in slow motion. Vary this until you like trying it without the jerking of the hands. Concentrate your mind on the biceps until you can get just one response to your efforts. This is the secret of all muscle control work. Once you can feel the muscles moving at your command, you get the feeling that you are winning. Until you get this feeling, it can be very hard work without any seemingly prospect of making the various muscle groups move at your command.

Do not stick tight to this position, but try it with your hands behind your head, as in Photo 24, or with your hands on top of your head, with the fingers loosely interlaced.

Exercise 33

Now go to the pectoral muscles. With the hands in front of the waist, make these muscles move about quickly and intermix this with a firm deliberate contraction. When this is done correctly, you will have a view of your pecs standing out like two pieces of rope, hollow underneath the protruding clavicles (collar bones) which make the trapezius muscles prominent. Practice this until you can get this effect with the hands apart.

This pose is in direct opposition to the next one, which is for the trapezius muscle, the big muscle which makes the slope from your head to your shoulders. When I was touring the theatres as a professional wrestler, this was the muscle that I carefully noted on my opponent. To me, it's development gave me an idea of his strength. . .

Exercise 34 – TRAPEZIUS

To get this control, immediately place your hands from in front to behind the buttocks, grasping a couple of fingers of one hand with the other hand, palms backward. Stand upright. Stoop a little with your shoulders and sink your head in towards your shoulders and force the head backwards. This should give the appearance of a full chest and the trapezius muscle on either side linked together. Whilst doing this, a pull on the hands will make the "traps" more prominent.

Exercise 35

You could now bring in your forearms. To get these under control, you will hold your arms outward and midway between your waist and your shoulders. Hold the arms slightly bent and grip your fists lightly, with palms upward. Grip fists tightly and turn your hands inward with a downward movement. This should make the appearance of a "swan's neck". Relax the grip, and tighten up again alternately, at the same time moving you hands towards your shoulders and try to work your hands in a circular movement from your wrists. The more you can bring your hands in towards your forearms, the better will you feel the effect of the control. Like the other controls, you should practice until you can do it without the gripping of the fists.

If you will turn around, you could now work on your shoulder muscles in general. . .

Start by taking the arms overhead as in Photo 7. When holding this position, you will reach a little higher by giving the hands a kind of wriggle at the same time try to pull those "lats" muscles behind the arms, (lattissimus dorsi) out a little. Move in alternate movements and bring your shoulders in towards your neck. This is a very important move, so do spend a little time to make the shoulder-blades (scapulae) spread outward. Pause slightly, then repeat the shrug with a little more effort. Now keep pulling hard at your hands and slowly lower your hands down to the crown of your head. Straighten the arms again. Do another shrug and this time lower one arm outwards. This will bring the other arm across the top of your head. Keep pulling. Return to the Photo 7 position. Another shrug, then lower the arm outwards. Still pulling, return to Photo 7 position, then lower the hands to the crown of the head. This will give you a chance to do the circular movement with the shoulders – and this is a movement that is greatly admired by Tony's audience.

Exercise 37

We can go from this down to the Triceps Control – Photo 14. This should be done with one hand holding the thumb of the other hand, although if you can do it with the fingers interlaced it will do. The idea with this is to make the triceps on each arm jump about simultaneously and alternately.

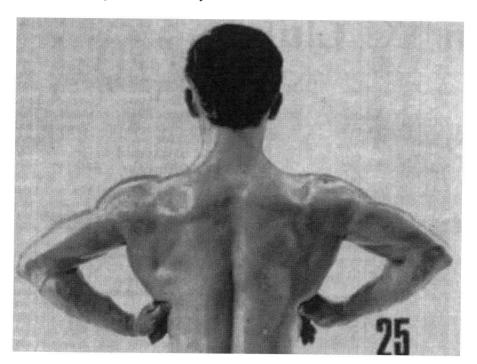

PART 7: MUSCLE CONTROL MOVEMENTS
FOR THE FIFTH MONTH
Exercise 38

Follow this by placing your hands on your hips, as Tony is holding his arms in Photo 25. The hands on the hips position is usually the best way to master this control. You will probably agree with me that Tony is able to perform many of the control movements a little different to others, (and here he places his hands higher on the body) and this is because he has spent so much time in arranging his routine to make that special appeal to his audience. Of course, you may be able to duplicate his movements. Later on, you will have a little exercising with a combination of moves to get a really pronounced effect.

Having placed your hands on your hips, press hard on your hips and push your shoulders in towards the sides of your head. This will give a hunched-up appearance. Now drop your shoulders and spread your elbows outwards, taking them slightly forward, and this should broaden your back as in Photo 25. Relax completely, then repeat. When you get the idea of this, you can place your hands on your hips and make a circular movement with the shoulders, taking them close to your ears, then backward and forward. One thing that you must concentrate on is to take your elbows backward, then forward whilst making this circular movement, and the elbows should be spread out to make a very wide sweep.

Whilst making this sweeping circular movement, you will be able to feel the scapulae in action. To get this favorably, you will spread your shoulders out as in Photo 26. As I mentioned earlier, it will take much practice to get sufficient control to do it with your hands held in the same position as Tony holds them. This is another proof of his wonderful control.

Whilst on the Lats and Scapula Controls, I should ask you to face a mirror and repeat these controls. This will have a marked effect if you will raise your chest and draw in your abdominals. The display of the lats looks very prominent from the front view.

Exercise 39 – THIGH, CALF AND KNEE CAP MOVING

With the front view of the legs, the knee cap should be moved up and down to bring the thigh muscles into action. To bring the calf muscles into action it would be necessary to raise the heel of one foot. This will relax the calf muscle, (gastrocnemius group), and by a slight movement of the heel, you could make the calf muscle jump about.

As mentioned before, all these control movements should be practiced until they can be done without a noticeable movement of the hands or feet.

Exercise 40 – BICEPS OF LEGS

Here is an exercise which will develop the biceps muscles of the legs – the biceps femoris group, or the hamstrings. These are the muscles at the back of the thighs.

Take the position as shown in Photo 19, leg bent backward. Keep the toes pointed and bring your heel in towards your thigh. If done correctly, you should feel the muscle in the back of your leg tightening up. If you get a painful feeling of cramp in this muscle, you should go easy with this movement. This is because the legs are unaccustomed with these movements.

When you get the legs ready to take a little more of this, you could vary the contraction movement by bending the leg with the foot inward instead of pointing forward. The more you lean forward and raise the leg higher, the more effect can be gained. When doing this leg bending, you should feel the muscles on the front of the leg getting fully stretched. These are the extensor muscles of the Quadriceps group – the rectus femoris, etc.

Whilst on the subject of the thigh muscles, it is possible to move one particular muscle in the middle of the front thigh without moving the kneecap.

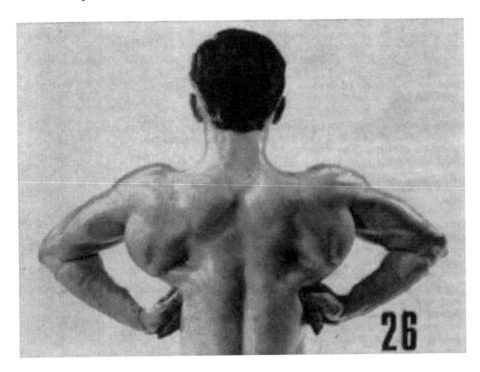

PART 8: ADVANCED CONTROLS
FOR THE FIFTH MONTH

We have now death with all the main muscle groups of the body with the exception of the isolation of the abdominal muscles – sometimes known as the "Rope", and this is a control most admired of all.

Exercise 41 – THE "CENTRAL ISOLATION"
or "THE ROPE"

The best method that I can suggest for quick results here is to lean forward with both hands on the edge of a table, with your feet about a yard or so away. Before you can get any feeling of this "rope", you must pull those abdominals in and force them out again, trying to get the abdomen in a little more each time. In fact, I have known it to be pushed in with the hands, but I always preferred doing it by concentration only.

When forcing the abdominals out again, there is a feeling which is very difficult to describe but, like many other outstanding feats, practice alone will produce it. But it might be advisable to check up on your feel and try a very slight alteration.

Take particular care in inhale and exhale before doing these abdominal movements. Do not expand the chest nor contract any other muscles.

On looking at Photo 27, showing Tony Holland performing the Abdominal Isolation, you will notice that he is doing it with his hands placed flat on his thighs. This again is an advanced method. You will find it much more helpful if you place your hands on the bottom of your abdomen, grasping the thumb of one hand with the palm of the body. You can try this whilst standing. You will need a droop of the shoulders to get a good effect. It must be practiced daily, because the abdominal muscles can lose their firmness.

Like other controls, it may take a long time and it may also seem to be an impossibility. I have known far too many pupils who have been disappointed with the lack of response but once you get the feeling that it is a possibility, you will be very delighted.

Forgive me for repeating some advice but some controls have such a distant appearance that a little encouragement and the truth without misleading is really necessary.

If you have done a fair amount of practice with Exercise 26, you should be able to make a reasonable attempt at this isolation control. I can assure you that it will take much concentration and practice, and the abdominals must be in really good condition to have any hope of making the Rope appearance. Like many other things which are difficult to achieve, it may surprise you to know the the first signs of feeling the success of it may come very unexpected. In fact, this can of "accidental success" is how many of the expert advanced controls are discovered. You must never despair nor get that inferior complex feeling of thinking that you will never do it.

I will now give you the performer's method of doing this feat. Stand upright, grasp the left thumb with the right hand, place the heels of your hands on the bottom of your abdomen – inhale, exhale. Raise your chest and expand it without inhaling. Let your shoulders come forward and draw the abdominal muscles inward with the idea of getting them inside your chest cavity. Try to forget about your abdominals, and press hard against your body with your hands, with a down towards the floor feeling. Now let your abdominal muscles fall down again. This should make a cavity on each side of the rectus abdominis muscles, hence the name "Rope".

It may be a good idea to check up on these points. Forget about any contraction of the muscles, because this could bring them down into a rubbing-board appearance. Do not bring the shoulders too far forward.

Before describing how I learnt this control, let me put your mind at rest again as regards to how Tony is showing the position. He is an expertly advanced performer and some other of his poses in this Course are the advanced work of the expert.

I would stand approximately a yard (36 inches) from a table – or similar article. Bend forward and place the palms of my hands on the table. This would enable me to get my abdominals well inward. I had a kind of forcing process when letting the muscles fall down again. It was a kind of squeeze and when I could feel the rope appearance, I would stand upright and try it the same way that the performers do it.

Yes, this is probably the most difficult and the most sought-after

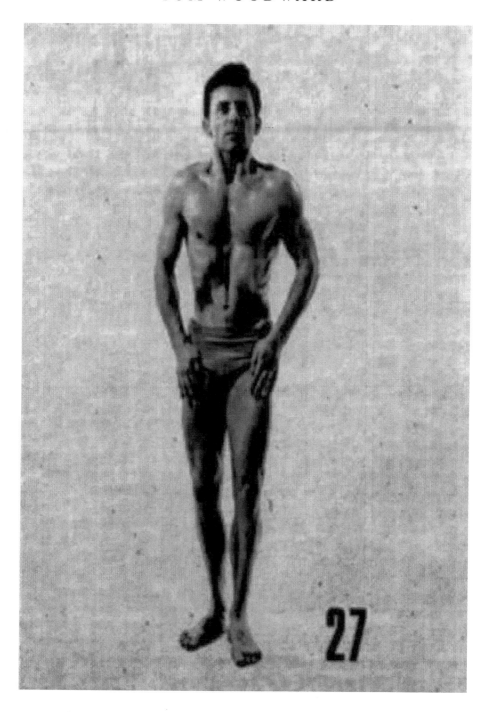

muscle control of all, with the exception of the one-sided isolation which I will describe later in the course.

PART 9: ADVANCED CONTROLS
Exercise 42 – THE ROLLING WAVES

Following the instruction for the "Rope" abdominal isolation control in the previous exercise, we can now try to get another kind of abdominal control, and this is one I like much better than the "rope". This exercise creates the impression of the transverse abdominis muscles appearing as rolling waves.

To get this effect, you should stand as in Photo 28. Draw in your abdomen as far as it will go, then let your muscles fall outwards, with the lower muscles falling out first. Then make them protrude, and draw them in again from the top of the group. In fact, the success of the control depends upon this alternate pulling-in and pushing-out movement.

After a few rolls, you could pause and show the abdominal group as in Photo 29. You have another good view of the abdominals as they should be in Photo 12.

Although the "Rope" abdominal isolation is much in favor, I really do prefer this abdominal control movement. When performed with the hands on the hips, as shown by Tony in Photo 29, it has a fascinating appearance. The idea is to stand as shown in this photograph and, as stated above, draw the abdominal muscles inwards and let them fall outwards again. After doing this a few times, you could try to make a kind of circular movement with the abdominals, letting them fall forwards as they come down, then drawing them back as far as possible when taking them inward and upward. Be content with doing one circular movement. Pause, then try another one. Making each one deliberate with the idea of showing the rolls of muscles. Add one repetition whenever possible, until you can do about half a dozen in smooth succession.

There are still two or three more advanced controls for the abdominals and neck with which I have yet to deal, but the instruction in this Course so far just about covers all the main groups of muscles which can come under control. I would now like to draw your attention again to Photo 26 and I somehow think that Tony Holland is the only muscle man I have seen to do this control, and a careful look at the photograph and at the position of the hands will give you an idea of what is needed to get this weird effect with the shoulder-blades (scapulae).

Part 10: MORE ADVANCED WORK

It was over sixty years ago when I first read a copy of Sandow's Magazine which included an article on Muscle Control, and although we have learnt a lot since that time about physical training, I still wonder if any of the present-day musclemen can bring more than one muscle-group into action at the same time. I would not put this beyond Tony Holland if he was asked to do it. I can still make the biceps of one arm, the triceps of the other, the thigh of one leg and the calf of the other move simultaneously, whilst in the seated position.

Let us look now at some more advanced resistance and contraction work for the neck muscles. These are clearly explained by looking at Photographs 30 and 31.

Exercise 43

Commence with the hands behind the head, as in Photo 30. Take the head backwards, at the same time resisting with your hands. This is primarily a neck strengthener, but when your head is well back, you can raise your elbows as high as possible and bring them inward, pulling on the rib muscles and raising your chest. Relax the chest and bring your head back to the starting point, pulling with your hands and resisting with your neck. Slowly continue the movement until your head is well forward as in Photo 31. If you have applied a fair amount of pressure, this should be sufficient for a start.

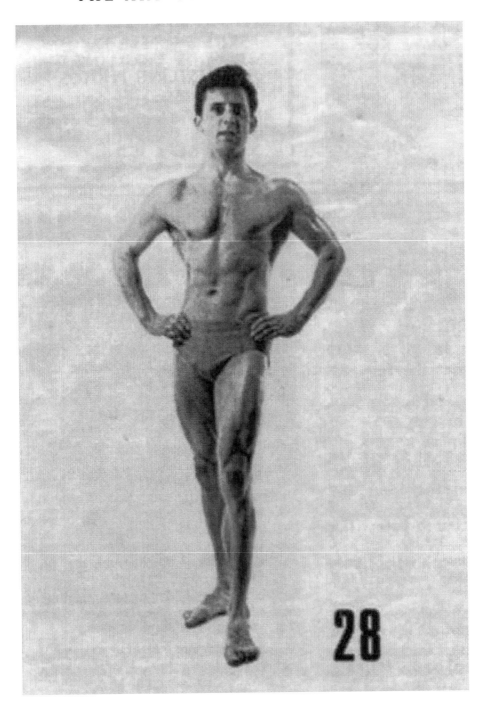

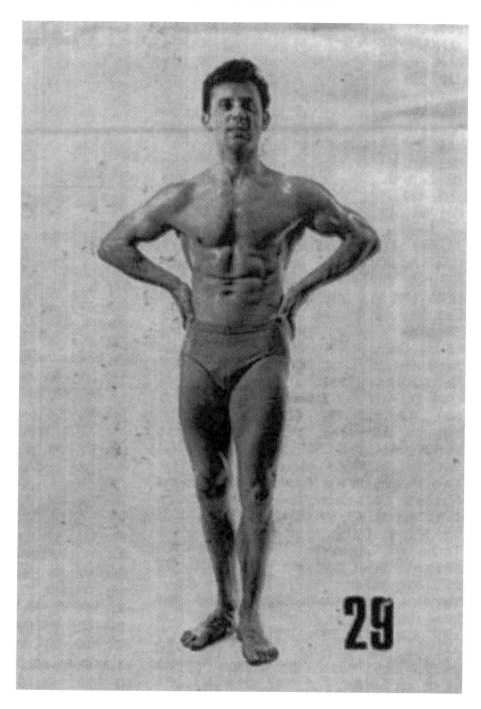

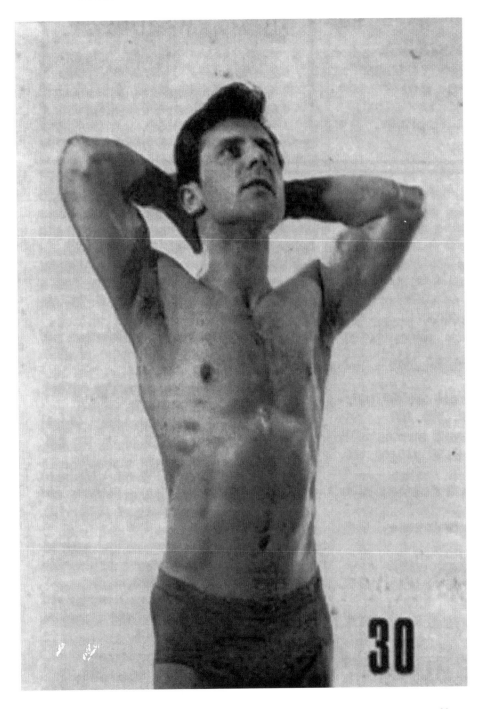

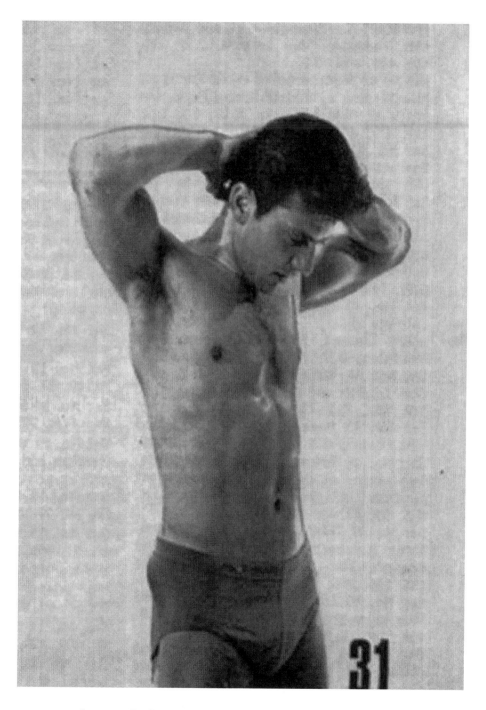

Exercise 44

Now for some contraction of the neck muscles. There is definitely one true saying about the physical make-up of any person interested in muscle development and it is that the neck is most important. A well-shaped neck adds to the general appearance even before the athlete is disrobed. If the neck is not developed to the same standard as the arms and chest it stands out like a blushing shame! You have had neck stretching and resistance movements, so you should be ready for a little contraction work.

This could be done whilst seated. Hold your head in its position, then try to shorten it by sinking it into your shoulders. Do this a couple of time only until the neck is able to take it. By all means do not be too eager and create a stiff neck. This could be very troublesome. When you are clearly satisfied that your neck is ready for some extra treatment, you could sink it into your body and move your head to each side alternately. Then make a circular movement, and then reverse the direction. Remember that you are trying to develop your neck, so do make the movements with this purpose in view.

For more old time classics of strength, visit:

STRONGMANBOOKS.COM

*Sign up on the website for a free gift and
updates about new books added regularly.*

Titles Available About and From All These Authors:

Arthur Saxon	William Blaikie
Bob Hoffman	Farmer Burns
Maxick	Monte Saldo
Eugen Sandow	Lionel Strongfort
George F. Jowett	Antone Matysek
Otto Arco	Harry Paschall
George Hackenschmidt	Louis Cyr
Thomas Inch	Alois Swoboda
Edward Aston	William Pullum
Bernarr MacFadden	Joe Bonomo
Earle Liederman	Siegmund Breitbart
Alan Calvert	Mighty Apollon
Alexander Zass	And Many More

Made in the USA
Lexington, KY
17 December 2013